WILDERNESS FIRST AID TECHNIQUES

A Complete Guide For Empowering Resilience Beyond Borders And Building Confidence In Critical Moments

WALTER ZYAIRE

DISCLAIMER

The information in this book is intended only for general informational purposes; it should not be used in lieu of professional advice or medical care. Since the author is not licensed to practice therapy, the information offered should not be used in place of the expertise, judgment, or guidance of qualified mental health or medical professionals. Readers are encouraged to consult therapists, medical specialists, or other qualified authorities regarding their particular situation and needs. The publisher and author disclaim all liability for any actions or decisions taken by readers based on the information in this book. Results may vary from person to person and this book's approaches, procedures, and strategies may not be suitable in all circumstances. Considering unique situations and consulting a qualified expert are essential when choosing the right course of action. Neither the publisher nor the author recommend or guarantee the efficacy of any therapy or treatment that is indicated in this book. Because the information is based on the author's research and understanding at the time of publishing, it could not reflect the most recent developments or practices in the treatment area. The publisher and the author both disclaim all liability for the accuracy, completeness, or use of the material in this book. Readers bear full responsibility for the decisions and actions they choose in light of the information presented in this book.

TABLE OF CONTENTS

ABOUT THE BOOK

The book "Wilderness First Aid Techniques" is essential reading for anyone hoping to gain the information and abilities needed to handle medical situations in the great outdoors. This extensive guide's main goal is to give readers a full grasp of wilderness first aid. It is intended for a wide range of readers, including hikers, outdoor lovers, professional guides, and rescue workers.

The book's explore the essential elements of wilderness first aid, including its definition, application, and guiding principles. These are essential skills to have. The significance of responding responsibly and ethically in emergencies is emphasized while legal and ethical considerations are also examined.

The book goes into deeper detail on fundamental anatomy and physiology, giving readers the ability to distinguish between normal and aberrant symptoms and indicators in a wilderness setting.

A large portion of the book is devoted to evaluating the conditions in the wilderness, with a focus on the importance of scene safety, size-up, and primary and secondary assessments. The book goes over a wide range of typical injuries and diseases that occur in the outdoors, from cuts and abrasions to heat-related illnesses and allergic reactions. Comprehensive information about the identification, management, and avoidance of these disorders is included in every section.

The thorough examination of first aid methods designed for use in wilderness situations forms the core of the book. The book offers a thorough manual on managing a variety of emergency scenarios, from CPR and rescue breathing to wound treatment, splinting, and shock management. In addition, the chapters on medical emergencies, evacuation and rescue, and the necessities of a first aid pack provide readers with the information they need to make wise choices in difficult outdoor circumstances.

Particular emphasis is paid to specifics, including sections devoted to psychiatric first aid, pet first aid, and wilderness first aid for kids. The variety of potential emergency scenarios in the wilderness is acknowledged by the inclusion of these themes.

The book concentrates on training and certification, directing readers toward official courses and certification courses that will improve their ability to provide wilderness first aid. All things considered, "Wilderness First Aid Techniques" is a priceless tool that provides a comprehensive awareness of, prevention for, and response to medical emergencies in the wide and unpredictably changing wilderness.

CHAPTER ONE

OVERVIEW OF WILDERNESS FIRST AID TECHNIQUES

WHY WILDERNESS FIRST AID IS SO IMPORTANT

The value of Wilderness First Aid (WFA) in the context of outdoor exploration and adventures cannot be emphasized. Enthusiasts who pursue the excitement of venturing into isolated and untamed environments invariably subject themselves to a plethora of possible hazards and crises. To effectively bridge the gap between standard first aid procedures and the particular difficulties posed by the erratic and frequently severe conditions of the environment, wilderness first aid is an essential skill set.

RECOGNIZING THE NEEDS OF WILDERNESS FIRST AID

Recognizing how wilderness first aid differs from traditional first aid is essential to understanding it.

Although first aid training at the basic level prepares people to manage injuries and emergencies in more controlled settings, wilderness first aid (WFA) expands this understanding to situations in which medical assistance can be hours or even days away. It includes an all-encompassing strategy that takes into account the surrounding conditions, scarce resources, and the requirement for adaptability when handling illnesses or injuries in the great outdoors.

DEFINITION AND EXTENT

The range of scenarios that adventurers may face in isolated areas is covered by the comprehensive breadth of Wilderness First Aid. WFA dives into the special difficulties provided by nature, from diagnosing and treating injuries brought on by contact with wildlife to handling environmental crises like hypothermia or heatstroke. It goes beyond the conventional medical approach by placing more emphasis on flexibility and adaptability to the current situation, where resources are limited and evacuation might not be possible right away.

IMPORTANT IDEAS

The concepts of independence and resourcefulness serve as the cornerstones of Wilderness First Aid. Practitioners are taught to consider the constraints of the wilderness setting but to put the patient's needs first. These guidelines consist of the three ABCs of wilderness first aid: being aware of one's surroundings, keeping a composed and assured demeanor, and acting quickly to tend to the sick or injured. Furthermore, a key component of WFA comprehends the principles of rating and classifying injuries according to their severity and possible impact on the patient's life.

A LEGAL AND ETHICAL PERSPECTIVE

The field of Wilderness First Aid is further complicated by ethical and legal issues. Those who have received WFA training may find themselves having to make important decisions with legal ramifications if they do not receive prompt expert medical care. Crucial components of WFA include knowing one's limitations, getting informed permission, and negotiating the legal environment when delivering care in remote locations. Furthermore, ethical issues arise when attempting to strike a balance between the patient's well-being and the preservation of the environment, underscoring the necessity of a sustainable and responsible method of providing medical care in remote areas.

Wilderness first aid is an essential set of skills for both professionals and outdoor amateurs. It is important not just because it can save lives in difficult situations but also because it can make people who go into the wilderness feel more responsible and prepared. The ability to recognize and use Wilderness First Aid provides a crucial safety net as we explore the wonders and unpredictable nature of the natural world, guaranteeing that the quest for adventure will always be exciting, safe, and sustainable.

CHAPTER TWO

ANATOMY AND PHYSIOLOGY BASICS

AN OVERVIEW OF THE SYSTEMS IN THE HUMAN BODY

The human body is a complex, networked system made up of many tissues and organs that cooperate to keep homeostasis. To appreciate the intricacy of physiological processes, one must have a general understanding of the systems that make up the human body. Eleven major systems make up the body, and each has a distinct purpose and job. The neurological, endocrine, circulatory, lymphatic, pulmonary, digestive, urinary, and reproductive systems are among these systems, as are the integumentary, skeletal, muscular, and nerve systems. Every system makes a distinct contribution to the person's overall well-being.

The integumentary system, which includes the skin, hair, and nails, helps to control body temperature and serves as a barrier against outside hazards.

In addition to offering structural support and safeguarding important organs, the skeletal system is where blood cells are formed. The muscular system, which is made up of muscles, supports and facilitates a variety of body activities.

The hormone-secreting glands that make up the endocrine system control several physiological functions, including growth, metabolism, and reproduction. The circulatory system, which is made up of the heart and blood vessels, moves waste materials out of the body and distributes hormones, nutrients, and oxygen throughout it. The lymphatic system supports immunological response and fluid homeostasis, assisting the body's defense against infections. Gas exchange is facilitated by the respiratory system, which includes the lungs and airways, and permits the intake of oxygen and the expulsion of carbon dioxide.

Nutrients from meals are broken down and absorbed by the digestive system, which supplies vital energy for body processes. The urinary system keeps fluid and electrolyte balance as well as gets rid of waste. Lastly, by aiding in the generation of progeny, the reproductive system guarantees the survival of the species.

TELLING A NORMAL SIGN FROM AN ABNORMAL ONE

It's critical to distinguish between normal and abnormal symptoms to evaluate and maintain a person's health. Physiological parameters that fall within the typical range for a healthy individual are referred to as normal signals. Vital signs are important markers of general health, and they include body temperature, heart rate, blood pressure, and breathing rate. Variations from these standards could indicate a medical condition.

Signs of abnormality can take many different forms, including discomfort, swelling, skin color changes, and mental state abnormalities.

Metabolic diseases may also be indicated by anomalies in laboratory test findings, such as blood glucose levels or lipid profiles. When these aberrations are identified, additional research and action are taken to find and address the underlying source of the irregularity.

Fostering health and quickly resolving possible problems require a thorough awareness of the systems of the human body as well as the capacity to distinguish between normal and abnormal indicators. This information serves as the foundation for healthcare practitioners' assessments, diagnoses, and treatments of a broad range of medical disorders, enhancing people's general health.

CHAPTER THREE

EXAMINING THE CIRCUMSTANCES

SCENE SECURITY

An essential part of emergency response is situation assessment, which entails using a methodical strategy to obtain data and make defensible conclusions. Scene safety, Size-Up, and Primary Assessment, and Secondary Assessment are the three main ideas in this procedure.

The priority in any emergency response is scene safety. Responders need to make sure the area is safe for them and any possible victims before they approach a scenario. Risks like fire, dangerous materials, or unfriendly people must be recognized and dealt with in a way. This first action lays the groundwork for efficient emergency response because it creates a safe setting, which protects responders' health and safety as they conduct further assessments and interventions.

SIZE-UP AND INITIAL EVALUATION

Understanding the extent and nature of an emergency requires taking the Size-Up and Primary Assessment procedures. Size-Up entails a fast and thorough assessment of the overall scene, taking into account variables such as patient count, potential risks, and resource availability.

Responders can create a basic plan of action for handling the problem in this step. The most seriously injured or unwell people's immediate requirements are the focus of the Primary Assessment that comes next. This entails evaluating the breathing, circulation, and airway (ABCs) and quickly attending to any life-threatening conditions. Size-Up and Primary Assessments are quick, comprehensive procedures that lay the groundwork for longer, more in-depth assessments later on.

SECONDARY EVALUATION

Secondary Assessment explores each patient's overall assessment in greater detail. After responding agencies have treated any life-threatening concerns during the Primary Assessment, they can go over the patient's wounds or illnesses in greater detail.

This includes taking vital signs, conducting a complete physical examination, and getting a thorough medical history. A more comprehensive assessment of the patient's state is provided by the Secondary Assessment, which helps determine the patient's priority for transportation and future interventions.

It is an essential step in ensuring that the response is customized to meet the unique requirements of every person impacted by the event.

A systematic approach to analyzing the situation in emergency response is formed by the ideas of Scene Safety, Size-Up and Primary Assessment, and Secondary Assessment taken together. Effective decision-making and interventions in dynamic and often tough settings are facilitated by prioritizing safety, comprehending the picture as a whole, addressing immediate life-threatening conditions, and performing thorough patient assessments.

CHAPTER FOUR

COMMON ILLNESSES AND INJURIES IN THE WILDERNESS

ABRASIONS, CUTS, AND SCRAPES

Cuts, scrapes, and abrasions are typical injuries in wilderness situations that can happen from hiking, climbing, or using tools. These injuries happen when friction, sharp objects, or rough surfaces cause damage to the skin's surface.

Preventing infections in the wilderness requires proper wound care. The wound can heal more quickly if it is cleaned with clean water and mild soap, treated with an antiseptic, and covered with a sterile bandage or dressing. For treating these small wounds in an outdoor environment, having a basic first aid kit on hand that includes sticky bandages, sterile dressings, and antiseptic wipes is essential.

BENDS AND TWISTS

Common injuries that occur in the outdoors are sprains and strains, which impact the muscles and ligaments, respectively. Activities involving abrupt movements, such as twisting an ankle on uneven ground or exerting yourself while carrying a large backpack, are common causes of these injuries. The cornerstones of treating these injuries are rest, ice, compression, and elevation (R.I.C.E.). Compression bandages, elevating the damaged limb, administering ice to minimize swelling, and resting the affected area can all aid in pain relief and speed up healing. To treat sprains and strains quickly, a compression bandage and an ice pack must be included in the backcountry first aid kit.

DISLOCATIONS AND FRACTURES

In the wilderness, falls, collisions and other traumatic events can cause fractures and dislocations. It is essential to identify the symptoms and indicators, such as deformity, swelling, and excruciating pain, to administer the proper first aid. It is crucial to immobilize the wounded limb as soon as possible with splints or homemade materials and to get professional medical attention. Maintaining fracture stabilization until more comprehensive medical treatment is available can be facilitated by keeping a small, light splint in the first aid bag.

DISEASES CAUSED BY THE HEAT

There is a considerable danger of heat-related illnesses in hot and muggy wilderness settings. Prolonged exposure to high temperatures and dehydration can cause conditions including heat exhaustion and heat stroke. Maintaining hydration, dressing in airy, light clothing, and taking pauses in the shade are examples of preventive strategies. When someone shows signs of a heat-related disease, such as heavy perspiration, weakness, nausea, or confusion, it's critical to get them into a cooler place, give them some water, and get medical help as soon as possible.

INJURIES CAUSED BY COLDS

Low-temperature exposure in wilderness environments can result in cold-related injuries like frostbite and hypothermia. Preventing these conditions requires staying dry, wearing appropriate clothing, and using insulation. It's critical to identify early indicators of cold-related ailments, such as shivering, disorientation, or numbness, to treat them quickly. Managing these illnesses requires avoiding future exposure to cold weather, as well as providing warm shelter, dry clothing, and warm liquids.

BITS AND STINGS

In the wild, encounters with animals, insects, or plants can cause stings and bites. Bite reactions from insects, snakebite injuries, and contact with poisonous animals can range from mild pain to severe reactions. Outdoor enthusiasts should always carry a snakebite kit, wear bug repellent, and be familiar with basic first aid for bites and stings.

It's important to get medical help as soon as possible for venomous bites or stings since some reactions can call for specialized antivenom or other medical care.

REACTIONS ALLERGIC TO

People may be exposed to allergens in wilderness settings, which can cause allergic reactions. Allergies to particular foods, plants, or insects can cause symptoms that range from a slight discomfort to life-threatening anaphylaxis. It is imperative for anyone with known severe allergies to always have an epinephrine auto-injector on hand. Managing allergic reactions in the wilderness requires being aware of the symptoms, which include breathing difficulties, swelling, or hives, and getting medical help right away. Furthermore, reducing the incidence of allergic episodes can be achieved by taking preventive steps and being aware of common allergens in the area.

CHAPTER FIVE

FIRST AID METHODS

RESCUE BREATHING AND CPR

Cardiopulmonary Resuscitation (CPR) is an essential first aid method for reviving people who are going into cardiac arrest. Maintaining blood flow and oxygenation to critical organs is the fundamental objective of CPR until a trained medical assistant arrives. Rescue breathing and compressions are the two main parts of CPR.

The goal of chest compressions is to forcefully and quickly push on the middle of the chest to force blood throughout the body. By tilting the head back and elevating the chin, rescue breathing, on the other hand, involves giving the person breaths. When done quickly and successfully, the combination of rescue breathing and compressions can save lives.

METHODS FOR DRESSING AND CARING FOR WOUNDS

Infection prevention and wound healing depend on proper wound care. It's important to start wound care by thoroughly washing the area with water and mild soap to get rid of any debris or bacteria. Using an antiseptic solution after cleaning reduces the possibility of infection. Selecting the right dressing is essential; the wound can be covered with adhesive bandages or sterile gauze pads. Applying direct pressure and elevating the affected leg can help control bleeding in cases of bigger wounds or severe bleeding until expert medical treatment is available.

IMMOBILIZATION AND SPLINTING

Splinting is a method for immobilizing fractured bones, broken limbs, or wounded joints to lessen discomfort and stop additional damage. Stabilizing the damaged area is the main goal of splinting while you wait for medical assistance.

It is imperative to immobilize the injured limb in situations of fractures or suspected fractures by constructing a splint out of items like boards, rolled-up newspapers, or even clothing. The splint can be fastened in place with straps or bandages. Immobilization is essential to avoid movement that can exacerbate the injury and put the patient at risk for further damage.

HANDLING SCALDS AND BURNS

Exposure to heat, chemicals, electricity, or radiation can cause burns and scalds. Cooling the injured region under running water for at least ten to twenty minutes is the first step in immediate first aid for burns. This aids in lowering the burn's warmth and easing discomfort. It's crucial to avoid using ice or extremely cold water since they can exacerbate tissue damage. To prevent infection, cover the burn with a clean towel or sterile, non-stick dressing when it has cooled. Severe burns must be seen by a medical practitioner right once since they can need specific treatment.

HANDLING THE SHOCK

A medical emergency known as shock can result from several traumatic circumstances, including serious injury or unexpected sickness. Unless it aggravates existing injuries, the first aid for shock entails keeping the victim warm, keeping them in a comfortable position, and gently elevating their legs. Reassurance and maintaining the person's composure can assist stop additional tension. To stop heat loss, cover the person with a blanket or warm clothing if at all possible. Anyone experiencing shock should get medical help right away because this condition frequently signals a serious underlying issue that needs to be evaluated and treated by an expert.

CHAPTER SIX

EMERGENCY MEDICAL CARE IN THE BACKCOUNTRY

HEART ATTACKS AND CHEST PAIN

Medical emergencies in the backcountry can present serious difficulties, therefore it's important to know how to react in different scenarios to protect people's health. Heart attacks and chest pain are dangerous disorders that need to be treated right away. Because it may be difficult to get emergency medical care in the wilderness, knowing basic first aid techniques is crucial.

A heart-related problem is frequently suggested by chest pain. It's critical to identify the signs of a suspected heart attack, which include severe chest pain, pressure, or discomfort that may spread to the arms, neck, or jaw. Sweating, nausea, or dyspnea may also be present in those who are exhibiting these symptoms.

It is necessary to act immediately, and if emergency responders are available, they should be called.

It is crucial to maintain the affected person's composure and encourage them to rest while they wait for medical assistance. Helping someone who carries medicine prescribed for angina, like nitroglycerin, to take it as directed can help reduce symptoms. Keeping an eye on vital signs and offering comfort might help maintain a more stable state of affairs until more extensive medical care is obtained.

HEART ATTACK

When a stroke occurs in the woods, quick thinking and action are required. Disrupted blood flow to the brain causes a stroke, which may result in neurological problems and possible brain damage. It's important to recognize the warning indications of a stroke, which include sudden numbness or weakness in the arm, leg, or face, especially on one side of the body; confusion;

difficulty speaking; and difficulties understanding speech.

 When one is suspected of having a stroke, time is critical. The affected person should be advised to relax, and emergency services should be called right away. While waiting for expert aid, it's crucial to keep an eye on the patient's vital signs, make sure their airway is unobstructed, and position them comfortably and stably.

CONVULSIONS

 In the wilderness, seizures may be frightening events. It's important to know how to react to ensure the safety of both the person having the seizure and the people helping them. It's crucial to make sure the individual experiencing a seizure is secure by gently assisting them to the ground and away from any potential dangers. One way to help avoid choking is to turn the person onto their side.

It's crucial to time the seizure since more than five minutes of seizures can necessitate immediate medical intervention. Since most seizures are self-limiting and go away on their own, it is important to maintain your composure. Following the seizure, it is advised to offer a quiet and comforting atmosphere, assist the individual in reorienting themselves, and see a medical specialist.

BREATHING PROBLEMS

In the wild, several things might cause respiratory discomfort, including respiratory infections, allergic reactions, or asthma episodes. For the right course of action to be taken, it is imperative to identify the symptoms of respiratory distress, which include breathing difficulties, wheezing, and a bluish tint to the lips or face.

Helping the person experiencing respiratory distress to settle into a comfortable position is critical; this is usually sitting up straight with a small forward inclination.

Assisting the person with the prescription inhaler can be helpful if they have one for an asthmatic or other medical condition. It's critical to keep an eye on the person's breathing, maintain composure, and seek emergency medical attention as needed when handling respiratory distress in the outdoors.

COMMUNICATION FOR EVACUATION AND RESCUE IN THE WILDERNESS

When it comes to wilderness rescue and evacuation, effective communication is essential. The reliability of traditional modes of communication may be compromised in these tough and remote locations. As a result, to stay in contact, rescuers and evacuees must resort to alternate means. In these situations, radios, satellite phones, and emergency beacons are often utilized equipment. While satellite phones guarantee communication in places without cellular coverage, radios allow team members and base camps to communicate in real-time. Emergency beacons, which include Emergency Position Indicating Radio Beacons (EPIRBs) and Personal Locator Beacons (PLBs), are essential tools for informing the authorities of the whereabouts of people who are in difficulty. Furthermore, signaling tools like whistles and signal mirrors are necessary for short-range communication, particularly in circumstances where distance or noise may make spoken communication challenging.

CONSTRUCTING EMERGENCY SHELTERS

Making appropriate shelters is a vital component in wilderness rescue and evacuation. The safety of both rescuers and evacuees depends on having a dependable refuge during inclement weather or unplanned delays. When deciding where to build a shelter, it is important to understand the climate and topography. Caves, overhangs, and thick foliage are examples of natural features that can offer some early concealment. If there are no natural possibilities, makeshift shelters can be built from readily available materials like branches, leaves, and even snow. Rescue packs frequently contain portable emergency shelters, such as tents and bivouac sacks. The insulation and weather protection that these shelters offer enhance the general safety and comfort of individuals taking part in the rescue and evacuation operations.

Emergency Signaling: Coordinating rescuers to locate individuals in need and facilitating a prompt and successful evacuation depend heavily on effective signaling. Visual cues, like colorful clothes or flags, are essential for improving visibility, particularly in heavily forested or mountainous areas.

In low visibility situations, rescuers can locate people with the aid of audible signals like whistles. Whistle blasts and light signals can be programmed to emit distinct patterns that indicate certain messages, negating the necessity for spoken communication. Signaling mirrors, flashlights, and even flare cannons can draw attention from a distance in low-visibility situations. Furthermore, knowing and using international distress signals—like SOS in Morse code—increases the likelihood of being detected and saved by passing planes or bystanders. Both rescuers and evacuees must receive training in appropriate signaling strategies to guarantee a well-coordinated and effective response in difficult wilderness environments.

CHAPTER SEVEN

ESSENTIALS FOR A FIRST AID KIT

PUTTING TOGETHER A COMPLETE FIRST AID KIT

To properly handle minor wounds and medical situations, a thorough first aid pack must be assembled. To start, choose a sturdy and handy container to store your items in. When creating the package, take into account the unique requirements of your home, including any medical issues or allergies. Put basic supplies like sterile gauze, adhesive bandages, adhesive tape, scissors, and tweezers in your kit. Add personal belongings such as prescription drugs, emergency contact details, and a basic first-aid guidebook.

A first aid kit's contents can change depending on what you need it for, where you're going, and how many people you need to help. Add supplies like blister treatment, insect repellent, and a small thermal blanket if you're an outdoor enthusiast.

Pet-specific items should be included if you have any pets. Make sure everything in your first aid kit is up to date and in good condition by periodically reviewing and replacing any used or compromised goods.

PRESCRIPTIONS & MEDICATION

Your first aid kit's prescription and pharmaceutical contents should be carefully chosen based on each patient's unique medical requirements. Incorporate necessary over-the-counter drugs such as analgesics, antihistamines, and antidiarrheal drugs. Make sure the kit has a sufficient quantity of prescription drugs if any family members need them. Medication should be kept in its original container with instructions labeled clearly, and expiration dates should be checked frequently.

It's critical to speak with medical experts about any possible drug interactions and customize the first aid pack for each member of your household based on their individual medical needs.

Additionally, think about keeping emergency supplies like epinephrine inhalers or injectors on hand if someone has severe allergies or long-term medical issues.

MAINTENANCE ADVICE

Maintaining your first aid kit regularly can guarantee that it works well in an emergency. Make routine inspections and supply replenishments at least once every six months. Throw away any expired drugs and things that appear worn out or damaged. To keep perishables like lotions and ointments from spoiling, rotate them.

Keep the first aid kit updated on any changes in the health state of household members. Examine and practice utilizing the kit's contents, paying particular attention to any new additions. You might think about enrolling in a basic first aid and CPR course to improve your abilities and understanding so that you can respond to emergencies more skillfully.

You can greatly improve your capacity to respond to a variety of medical situations by devoting time and effort to assembling a thorough first aid kit that includes drugs and prescriptions customized to meet specific health needs and putting routine maintenance procedures in place.

CHAPTER EIGHT

PARTICULAR POINTS TO REMEMBER

CHILDREN'S WILDERNESS FIRST AID

Specialized training is required for Wilderness First Aid for Children to handle medical emergencies and accidents that could arise in outdoor environments. Children's physiology and size necessitate special considerations when providing wilderness first aid. Responders must modify their strategy in these situations to interact with and care for young patients. It is critical to identify and treat particular juvenile medical issues, such as allergic reactions or respiratory distress.

Children receiving first aid in the wilderness should be trained in addressing typical outdoor injuries including cuts, bug bites, and fractures, as well as doing CPR that is appropriate for the child's age. Additionally, in outdoor first aid scenarios, it is critical to comprehend the psychological effects of emergencies on kids and use techniques to keep them calm and interested.

PET FIRST AID IN THE WILDERNESS

Wilderness First Aid for Pets recognizes that medical crises can arise in outside contexts for animals as well. To guarantee the pet's well-being, responders need to be taught to spot symptoms of distress and give the right treatment. This could entail treating wounds, providing basic first aid, and managing conditions like heatstroke, dehydration, or toxin exposure. Using makeshift instruments and supplies to make bandages or splints is another aspect of wilderness first aid for animals.

To learn about the health history and any pre-existing issues of the animal, veterinarians must communicate effectively with pet owners. In wilderness environments, timely and appropriate care can make a big difference in a pet's outcome, just like it can with human first aid.

FIRST AID IN PSYCHOLOGY

Giving people affected by traumatic events quick access to emotional and psychological support is the goal of psychological first aid, a crucial component of emergency response. This idea is not just applicable in wilderness settings; it is especially important in circumstances where people could be subjected to the natural stresses of life or unanticipated catastrophes in isolated places. To assist people in coping with the immediate aftermath of a disaster, psychological first aid entails active listening, empathetic support, and practical assistance. Responders must be educated to see warning indications of distress, reassure people, and put them in touch with the right people or resources for additional mental health care. It is much more important to provide prompt and attentive psychological first aid in wilderness settings since the isolation and difficult surroundings might worsen psychological stress.

CHAPTER NINE

INSTRUCTION AND CERTIFICATION

COURSES ON WILDERNESS FIRST AID

Training programs in wilderness first aid are vital for providing people with the knowledge and abilities needed to handle medical crises in isolated and outdoor environments. The specific difficulties and situations that can occur in wilderness settings, when access to qualified medical treatment may be restricted, are the focus of these courses. If emergency medical assistance is not available, participants in Wilderness First Aid Courses acquire the skills necessary to evaluate and treat wounds and diseases, prioritize care in difficult circumstances, and make wise judgments.

The emphasis on creativity and inventiveness in Wilderness First Aid Courses is one of its main features. These courses enable participants to modify their knowledge and abilities to fit the unique conditions of the environment, in contrast to typical first aid training.

This covers treating environmental problems like hypothermia or dehydration as well as injuries like sprains and fractures. To help participants develop a sense of independence and fortitude in the face of hardship, they are also taught how to improvise medical instruments and make use of accessible materials.

PROGRAMS FOR CERTIFICATION

Participants in wilderness first aid certification programs receive official acknowledgment for their ability to handle medical emergencies in outside environments. These internationally recognized certificates are frequently provided by respectable organizations. Assessments of theoretical knowledge and practical skills are usually part of the certification process. A person who completes the certification program demonstrates that they have complied with the requirements set forth by the certifying authority and are qualified to administer first aid in wilderness settings.

Programs for certification cover more ground than only the technical side of first aid. They also impart a deeper comprehension of risk management, emergency communication techniques, and the value of collaboration. This all-encompassing method guarantees that trained personnel not only have the essential medical knowledge but can also make wise decisions under duress and cooperate in difficult situations.

Additionally, a wide range of people are served by Wilderness First Aid Courses and Certification Programs, including adventure guides, forestry professionals, and search and rescue workers in addition to outdoor lovers. The knowledge and abilities gained from these programs are beneficial to anyone who spends time in isolated locations and helps to build an atmosphere of readiness and safety in outdoor communities.

Certification programs and wilderness first aid courses are essential parts of being ready for anyone going into the great outdoors. The integration of practical instruction, theoretical understanding, and official certification guarantees that people are prepared to manage medical emergencies in remote areas, enhancing the general security and welfare of participants as well as the communities they interact with.